Praise for
5 Things to Know for Successful and Lasting Weight Loss

In this quick-reading, common-sense book, Fran tells her own success story, which she has continued through today. She demonstrates what commitment and perseverance can do to conquer obesity and allow a person to live a rich, healthy life.

–George B. Cheponis, M.D.

Fran DiVecchio feels that losing weight is a mental challenge, not just a physical task. She warns that we should not just lose weight for some short-term wish, but rather keep in mind our long-term goal of permanent weight loss. She considers herself an "uncommon person" who is able to "put off instant gratification for a larger goal."

–Paula S. Youngdahl, M.D.

We all talk about losing weight, and we all know how to lose weight. But when we try, many of us, time after time, still lose focus and fail. This is a different story, a true story of how one woman won the battle. Fran succeeded by always remembering her true goals: weight loss and, more importantly, maintenance. She stopped dreaming about it and took control of her life to drop the unwanted pounds.

–Jayne Fincke, R.Ph.

After reading multiple "how-to" books and diet advice books, I have finally found a volume that is both inspiring and practical. Coupled with [Fran's] story are inspirational ideas that can motivate for many other difficult journeys. As she tells her story, you the reader become inspired to make similar lifestyle changes too.

–Mrs. E. G. Pellathy

If you want a sensible philosophy of how to become an agent of change in your own life for health's sake, this is it! Definitely, this book is a must-read for anyone who wants to move forward!

–Dr. Gene Dangelo, Educator

5 Things to Know for Successful and Lasting Weight Loss

5 Things to Know for Successful and Lasting Weight Loss

By Fran DiVecchio

TRADE PAPER
PRESS

Turner Publishing Company
200 4th Avenue North • Suite 950
Nashville, Tennessee 37219
(615) 255-2665

www.turnerpublishing.com

5 Things to Know for Successful and Lasting Weight Loss

Library of Congress Cataloging-in-Publication Data

DiVecchio, Fran.
 5 things to know for successful and lasting weight loss / by Fran DiVecchio.
    p. cm.
 ISBN 978-1-59652-558-0
1. Weight loss--Popular works. 2. Nutrition--Popular works. 3. Physical fitness--Popular works. I. Title.
II. Title: Five things to know for successful and lasting weight loss.
 RM222.2.D593 2010
 613.2'5--dc22
                          2009040413

Printed in China

10 11 12 13 14 15 16 17—0 9 8 7 6 5 4 3 2 1

I dedicate this book to my family—thank you.

All our dreams can come true,
if we have the courage to pursue them.

~Walt Disney

This one step—choosing a goal
and sticking to it—changes everything.

~Scott Reed, Author

Contents

*The only place where success comes before work
is in a dictionary.*

~Vidal Sassoon

You have to train your mind like you train your body.

~Bruce Jenner

Acknowledgments

"The future belongs to those who believe in the beauty of their dreams."
—Eleanor Roosevelt

There are so many people who helped me to believe in the beauty of my dream and have been supportive of this project. Without their encouragement, the idea of writing this book would have stayed in my head. In particular, I want to thank the following people:

My family: My parents and brother cheered me on every step of the way. The three of you have always been, and continue to be, my strongest support system. I love you.

Many thanks to the team of talented people at Turner Publishing Company, who helped me bring this book to fruition. My endless appreciation goes to my editor, Christina Huffines, who gave the book the final professional polish needed before it went to print. Thank you for being so detail-oriented, helpful, and supportive. Thanks to Rachel Joiner for guiding me through the initial stages of the publishing process, Mike Penticost for the awesome cover design, and Michael McCalip for helping with the entire process.

Jennifer, my cousin, for helping to write and kitchen-test every recipe in this book.

Keith (Kip) Richeal and Emmy Pellathy for the hours they spent helping me to achieve this goal. Emmy was instrumental in breaking the book down into chapters and helping me to restructure and reorganize the book.

Dr. Eugene M. Dangelo, Ph.D. Gene always encouraged me to keep going no matter how many times I wanted to pull the plug on this project. So many times he told me, "Don't give up. Remember, *Gone with the Wind* was rejected 39 times before it got picked up."

Jennifer McGuiggan, my Pittsburgh editor, who gave my manuscript the professional polish it needed before the acquisitions process. She guided me gently through the entire process and was able to bring out the best in my writing. Every time I started to stress out and thought about quitting this project, she immediately put a smile back on my face with the same three words, "Fran, calm down!" Jennifer's editing skills helped me to remain confident that we could make this book the best it can be.

Kelly Frey, morning news anchor from WTAE-TV Channel 4 Action News in Pittsburgh.

Debbi Casini Klein: Words cannot express my gratitude for your time, expertise, and support.

Barbara Miller: You have been a wonderful mentor.

Heidi Herholz: Thanks for your photography expertise.

The medical experts who were giving of their time: George B. Cheponis, M.D., Paula S. Youngdahl, M.D., Jayne Fincke, R.Ph., and Dan Dimpel, PharmD.

WTAE-TV Channel 4 Action News Pittsburgh, WQED-TV Channel 13, *Personal Best Magazine*, and the *Jennifer Antkowiak Show*.

My friends Megan Burke and Lynn Lucci, who read many revisions of the manuscript.

Foreword

Being a personal fitness trainer for over twenty years, I have made a living working in the company of people who want to lose weight. I have seen many weight-loss books, gadgets, and ideas come and go. Every one of them is the "it thing" at the time, the magical formula for weight loss and happiness.

I met Fran DiVecchio after she had already lost her extra weight. She works out at the health club where I am a trainer, and we began talking one day. This small, enthusiastic woman walked up to me with a question about exercise intensity. I had seen Fran in the club for a while—she was the one who brought a little lunch box with her and had a bowl of cereal after her early morning workout.

When you first meet someone, you assume that they have always looked like they do. One day I sat down with Fran during her mid-workout "cereal break." She is a very private person, but she began telling me about her weight-loss journey.

Fran is also a small person, just over five feet, so I could not imagine loading another 100 pounds onto her tiny frame. We talked about the unhappiness and frustration that comes with being overweight. She told me that she believes that weight loss is mainly a cerebral pursuit—a philosophy which I agree with 100 percent.

When I begin working out with new clients who want to lose weight, I ask them to go home and get out a sheet of paper. I explain that the most important thing they can do to achieve their goals has nothing to do with me, or even with exercise. I ask them to come up with three things that are keeping them from being successful at losing weight. I want them to be very specific. Simply saying "I eat too much" isn't going to cut it. I'm looking for more specific behaviors.

Everyone's three things are different, and there

may be more than three, but they have to start somewhere. Most people fight this assignment. "Aren't you going to give me a body-fat test?" they ask. Or, "Aren't we going to do sit-ups, or get on a treadmill, or talk about carbs?" Sometimes they want to know, "Where's my list of things that I can eat!?" "Not so fast," I tell them. "What are your three things?"

Fran succeeded in her weight-loss journey because she understood the mental aspect of pursuing her goal. Unfortunately, there is no magic formula for weight loss. How easy my job would be if there was! (Then again, maybe I wouldn't have a job!)

Those who identify and take personal responsibility for their weight-loss goals are more likely to achieve them. Many people want to give me that responsibility. "Tell me what to do," they say. It doesn't work that way. This is not to say a person should not seek guidance—quite the contrary. But soak up the information like a sponge, then run with it. What people do outside the gym has more impact on their weight than what they do in the gym.

Weight loss begins in your mind. You are what you think about. Why did you get fat in the first place? What is keeping you fat? What behaviors do you repeat over and over again? Or what do you not do? What do you think about while you eat? Why is change so hard for you in this area of your life? What need are you satisfying while keeping destructive behaviors alive? Most people never give any of this a thought. But Fran thought about it a lot. And then she did the tough part. After identifying the things that kept her stuck, she decided to slowly change those existing behaviors. She began to move in the right direction.

I'm not saying that losing weight is easy, but the process is not complicated. Can you give up your old weight-loss dialogue, the very way you approach the whole process? The one you have used over and over and over again?

It takes a white-hot passion to change who you are in relation to food and your activity level. This method isn't something you can find outside of yourself; it is very personal. Fran understood this mind-body connection. She understood that this was a very personal challenge, one she needed to be responsible for. She needed to get to know herself first. By doing that, she has kept off her excess weight for many years.

The decision to lose weight and get healthy can be a new, fantastic adventure for you. It's a path that very few people are willing to explore, but one that is well worth the effort.

—Susan Waldrop, Personal Trainer/Coach

Introduction

*"You're not going to succeed by just doing what is
required; it's going to be the little extra."*
  —Herb Brooks, U.S. Hockey Team and NHL Coach

You picked up this book because you felt that it
held something within its pages that was for
you. Indeed it does. This book holds discoveries that
can be of value to every human being. It is a treasure
trove of gems that some people may take a lifetime
to find. Here, they are set forth for you in one place.
Read on to see how these gems have helped me, and
how they may help you as well.

   This is a tale of both loss and triumph. This is a
book about how I lost 100 pounds and have kept it
off for over twelve years. This book of five simple

things to help you lose weight is not a how-to book or a book of "diet secrets." Instead, it is about how my personal journey can help you set—and keep— your own goals. This is a book about decision making and personal responsibility.

I suspect that many of you are reading this because you want to lose weight. My hope is that once you understand the basic success principles we'll explore in these pages, you will apply them to all areas of your life, wherever you need to set a goal and stick to it. The success principles I used to achieve and maintain my weight loss are nothing new in the world of motivational books. The real self-help secret is that you have to help yourself. You will see that I am an ordinary person—just like you—who had a fervent desire to accomplish a goal.

I used these success principles to turn my desires into real goals and to remain passionate about them. Maintenance requires discipline and enthusiasm, which must come from our passion and emotion.

Without those, we lose the motivation to stay the course. But if you learn to set real goals and persevere, you will be unstoppable.

Olympic Inspiration

I like to picture feats of goal setting and accomplishments in terms of an Olympic competition. Although I am no Olympic athlete, I like to find ways that I am similar to one. Not many athletes get to participate in the Olympics. Still, anyone who sets goals and overcomes the many difficulties in achieving these goals can become "uncommon." I use that term in the sense that the late Herb Brooks did when he coached the inexperienced U.S. hockey team to victory in the 1980 Olympics against the Soviet Union powerhouse team. In *Miracle,* the movie depicting that historical event, Brooks's character told his players, "This cannot be a team of common men, because common men go nowhere. You have to be uncommon." In other words, it takes uncommon fortitude to set and achieve goals in any situation.

The methodical pursuit of a goal and the struggle to succeed against multiple obstacles defines "uncommon." And while this is challenging, we can all become uncommon even as we pursue common goals. If you can be undeterred by failure and systematically pursue your golden dreams like Olympians pursue their gold medals, you will share that uncommon quality.

You may not have athletic dreams of winning a gold medal, but surely you have "gold medal" dreams. Do you dream of losing weight and being healthier? Do you long for a life in which you can climb a set of stairs without getting winded? Or perhaps you'd like to fit into your old college jeans or wear a bathing suit in public without feeling embarrassed. These dreams may not sound as big as the Olympics, but they're a big deal to you. To you, achieving those dreams would be golden, right?

My goal was to lose weight, a very common desire. I have learned to accept the need for exercise, and people often mistakenly think that I have a frustrated desire to be an athlete. I do not. I don't exercise for athletic competition or achievement, but for the sense of accomplishment—of achieving a goal that I have set for myself. I admire the level of commitment that Olympians exhibit during their training and competitions. It is that type of uncommon commitment that fuels me to stay focused on my own weight-loss goals. Common people do not compete in the Olympics and win gold medals. Common people do not set regular goals and work to achieve results. Uncommon people do these things.

I am a living example that ordinary people can celebrate uncommon victories over the ordinariness that keeps most of us bound to our old habits. I hope that by sharing my story I can keep you from making some of the same mistakes I did. Maybe we can become uncommon together.

As I strive to stay uncommon in my weight-loss goals, I have gained confidence to become uncommon in other areas of my life. Just look at the book in your hands! I'd never written a book before. I never even dreamed of the possibility! Yet now that I have achieved my goal of weight loss and maintenance, I am excited to tell my story. As you read my insights on successful weight loss and maintenance, I hope you will be inspired. I want you to become an uncommon person who can focus on a goal, make the commitment, and take the necessary actions to achieve this goal.

The five success principles in this book on achieving permanent weight loss have worked for me, but they are not a substitute for the advice of medical professionals. Before beginning any new health or weight-loss program, you should speak with a nutritionist, doctor, or other medical professional.

In order to achieve these goals, we first have to talk about the difference between a desire and a goal.

The 5 Things

You can never cross the ocean unless you have the courage to lose sight of the shore.

~Christopher Columbus

Whatever the mind can conceive and believe, it can achieve.

~Napolean Hill

— 1 —

Success Principle #1:
Change Desires into Goals

~ 1 ~

Success Principle #1:
Change Desires into Goals

"A journey of a thousand miles must begin with the first step."

—Lao Tzu

Desiring something and actually setting out to have it are radically different. We all have desires, wishes, and dreams. That is our common condition. What is uncommon is being able to set out on a path to fulfill those desires. Every journey, no matter how long, begins with the first step. But it's not enough to simply start walking. Your journey must have a destination; otherwise, each step could lead you in the wrong direction or end up as just marking time. Action without a definite direction, without a specific goal in sight, is action without purpose. Vaguely wishing for something is not the same as setting a goal. Even fervent desire and constant action are not enough to achieve results. These are ordinary responses to our desires. What we need are uncommon responses to achieve results. We need to turn our desires into goals.

Taking Responsibility

Over twelve years ago, at five feet one inch tall and 220 pounds, I was an ordinary person with a dream. I dreamed of losing weight, but lacked the energy and motivation to move away from my habits and pursue the dream. I considered myself a fairly active person, but in reality I never took the time to exercise, not even a ten-minute walk a few times a week. I was locked in a food prison of overeating, inactivity, and weight gain.

I didn't have a real weight problem until I went to college. Four years of commuting and unhealthy eating led to an extra 100 pounds on my petite frame. I went from a size 8 to a size 10, and then to a 12 and a 14. I eventually maxed out at a size 22. Year after year I watched the number on the tag increase while my choices for fashionable clothing decreased. It was painful to be 21 years old and wearing a size 22, shopping in the women's section while my friends still fit into the junior sizes. My mom and I would go shopping until the mirror reduced me to tears. This was not how I wanted to live, but I felt trapped by my habits, locked in my comfort zone. At that time, I did not fully realize the extent to which I controlled my own food consumption. I was never an emotional eater and didn't eat in response to frustration and sadness. But I was still not in control of my eating.

For example, in my twenties, my friends and I would often go to a movie and then end up at a 24-hour restaurant on a Saturday night. We would take up a table for a couple of hours, talking and having a good time. We actually just needed a place to hang out, so everyone just ordered something to drink. I always thought that our server must be frustrated with us for taking up her table without placing orders that would generate a decent tip. So I was always the first one to order some food. And because I was thoughtless about my choices, I always chose some sort of deep-fried appetizer.

Looking back and analyzing the situation, I realize there was more going on than me just feeling embarrassed for my table of friends. Beyond that, I was rationalizing my own desire for something to eat. Either way, I allowed external factors to control my eating habits. Plus, I was making a comfortable choice. Sure, I wanted to lose weight, but I liked fried foods and was used to eating them. At the time, I didn't see the event in an analytical way. I had the desire to lose weight but had not set the *goal* of weight loss.

Now I can see that I was the one who ordered and ate the food. My friends didn't make me do it. A grumpy waitress didn't make me do it. It was my decision. In order to lose weight, I had to learn to take responsibility for my food decisions. I couldn't just wish away the calories, or excuse them because I was having a good time with my friends. I had to create the goal of making wise eating choices, and then realize that it was up to me to attain that goal. (I continue to enjoy the company of my friends, but now I incorporate wiser food decisions than before. Changing my decisions about food doesn't mean I have to change everything.)

Setting Goals

It seems like the topic of weight loss is everywhere, from workplace conversations to bookstore shelves to the evening news. Everyone, from the housewife next door to the glamorous celebrity on the cover of a magazine, wants to be slim. The rich and famous often resort to extraordinary or invasive means to create their version of "the perfect body." Despite our culture's craze for being thin, achieving permanent weight loss remains only a desire for so many people. By staying stuck in our common habits, our dreams never become goals and thus never become realities.

Until I could change my desire into an achievable goal, I could not lose weight. Now I have obtained a height-appropriate weight and have maintained that weight—with a few minor setbacks—for over twelve years. How did I do this? It was a long and sometimes arduous journey, but I learned that weight loss is unachievable as a *desire*. In order to be achievable, weight loss has to become a goal.

What's the difference? Wishes, desires, and dreams are short-term "feel-good" strategies that can undermine serious achievement. Goals are long-term commitments that are achieved with systematic analysis and motivation. Uncommon people think in terms of goals. Turning a desire into an attainable goal requires certain principles that we can all put into practice. Let's go back to the analogy of being an Olympic athlete to find out how to turn our golden dreams into gold-medal goals.

Writing Down the Dream

"It's a dream until you write it down, and then it's a goal," said Bill Toomey, a decathlon Olympic gold medalist. What does it mean to write down your dream? It means to fix your desires permanently, to focus them, and to remove the distractions and clutter that often surround wishes and desires. When you write something down you must be specific.

Here's an example:

Desire: "I want to lose weight."

Goal: "I want to lose five pounds by the end of the month."

A goal is measurable and has a specific end result. Without concrete reference points, how can you tell if you are moving toward your goal? How will you know if you've reached it? By setting specific goals, we can see if we are making progress.

It's a good idea to take this idea of "writing down your dream" literally. Turn your dream into a goal and put it on paper. That way, you are less likely to forget it. By reminding yourself of it over and over again you can stay focused on the goal. So writing down your dream is really writing down your goal. It's creating something outside of yourself by capturing the dream in words. A dream exists only within your own mind, whereas a goal is outside of yourself, like a destination at the end of a road.

When I first started to lose weight, I wrote down very modest and attainable goals such as, "I will lose five pounds next month." I even wrote down the steps that would get me to that goal: "I will have three small meals a day for the next week," or "I will not eat any fried foods this week." Another way I stay focused on maintaining my weight loss is by using images. I keep photos of me from before and after my weight loss on the door of my refrigerator. Every time I open the fridge door, I am reminded of my goal: to maintain my desired weight.

Beyond athletic talent, Olympic athletes must possess the key component for success: mental preparation. Paavo Nurmi, a Finnish runner who won nine gold medals at the Olympic Games from 1920 to 1928, said, "Mind is everything. Muscle—pieces of rubber. All that I am, I am because of my mind." The same is true with any other endeavor, including weight loss. After choosing a goal, you must be prepared to achieve it through mental preparation. This leads us to the second success principle, which is all about your mind.

~ 2 ~

Success Principle #2:
Identify How You Got Here

~ 2 ~

Success Principle #2:
Identify How You Got Here

"Never live in the past but always learn from it."
                                                    —Anonymous

I want you to understand that for a long time, I didn't look at the reasons I was overweight. I'm not talking about the obvious reasons of eating too many calories and exercising too little. I'm talking about the underlying issues. Once I could pinpoint the reason I allowed myself to tip the scales at 220 pounds, I turned my desires into goals, reclaimed my life, and dropped the weight.

Everyone has a story full of high and low points. As you read mine, think about your own story and how it has shaped your choices.

My Story

I come from a very traditional Italian-American family. My dad was a steel worker for Jones and Laughlin Steel Corporation, but his real passion was his garden. That man had more gardening tools than most home and garden stores. When he wasn't working one of three different shifts at the steel mill, he spent summers in the garden. He believed that his own vegetables were more nutritious than what we could buy at the store. He worked hard for what he loved. "Fran, that's one thing—work never goes out of style," he told me. Years later I drew on his example and intensive work ethic to free myself from being overweight.

Like many women in her generation, my mom stayed home to raise me and my brother. If there was an Olympic event for cooking, she would be a gold medalist. She is a fantastic cook and always prepared very balanced and nutritious meals for us, even though I didn't always know it or appreciate it as a kid.

The lunches she packed me for school included sandwiches made with roasted red peppers, olive oil, and garlic—foods that are well-known today for being healthy. But kids don't know any better, and my classmates used to make fun of my lunch because the olive oil dripped onto the paper bag. Other kids teased me, saying I was poor because I couldn't afford a cafeteria lunch. I wanted to burst into tears when they said those things, but I wouldn't give them the satisfaction.

Still, one day I'd had enough. By the afternoon dismissal bell, I couldn't wait to get home to tell my mother about those mean cafeteria bullies. When I complained about being mistreated, she said: "Fran, those kids aren't using the brains that they were born with." She told me that they were just jealous.

My defining moment came the very next day in the cafeteria. Again the bullies started up: "Hey poor girl! You have the wet lunch bag again." I mustered up the courage that my mother had given me the night before, held my head up high, and said,

"You're just jealous of my homemade lunch. Anybody can just buy a lunch."

What I didn't realize at the time was that my mom was cultivating my self-worth and helping me to develop a tenacious personality from a young age. Along with my dad's work ethic, I would need these personality traits years later when I faced my weight-loss goal.

Like all good big brothers, my brother Gino took great pleasure in picking on me as a kid. He chased me around the house with spiders and generally harassed me. As an adult, Gino is very supportive of my efforts—in his own big brotherly way. He's always liked to play devil's advocate with me, which turns out to have made me a stronger person.

At Thanksgiving dinner in 1995, just five months after I started my weight-loss journey, my mom said, "Fran, I'm so proud that you've taken off thirty pounds. Keep going." Gino looked up from his plate of food and said, "Just wait until she gains it back!" At that moment I thought that Gino was being a jerk.

But I realized that his jokes were meant to support me during a difficult time. Because Gino was egging me on, I was more determined to stick to my goal. All in all, my personal background has helped me to remain confident in knowing who I am, even when I was hurt by how others viewed me when I was overweight.

Looking Inside

The second success principle of losing weight—looking at how you got here—must happen in conjunction with the first success principle of changing your desire into a goal. Many people attempt to lose weight without looking at the reasons they are overweight. I did this for a long time. While it's possible to reach your goal this way, more often than not, you will gain every pound back—plus some. I did this for twelve years until I took a look inside.

The reason that I was overweight for so many years is that I made everything except me a priority.

I was absent in my own life. During that time I was busy going to college and then working full-time while studying for a master's degree. I didn't take time to take care of myself. If I had honored myself, I wouldn't have gained so much extra weight. Identifying why I allowed myself to gain 100 pounds in the first place allowed me to get off the roller coaster ride for good and reclaim my life. The biggest injustice in this whole process was effectively losing twelve years of my life. And that's time that nobody can ever get back. I was trapped in a vicious cycle of weight loss and weight gain. But once I made myself a priority, I could take the steps necessary to free myself.

Taking care of yourself by exercising and eating the right kinds of foods is a *choice* that you make daily.

The choices we make impact us from the time we're kids. For example, I've always loved good food, especially my mom's Italian delicacies. Each December, she makes holiday biscotti. As a kid, I ate handfuls of these tasty treats. My mom often told me I was eating too many, but as soon as she went downstairs to get more ingredients, I sneaked a few more.

Looking back, I can see that I was doing what all kids do—enjoying sweets! But at the same time, I also see that I started a habit that I would have to lose. I was letting food dictate my actions. Our actions are indicative of who we are and should not be controlled by outside forces. The first biscotti tastes the same as the second or third. I realized that the taste of the biscotti should not dictate the quantity that I eat. I now see that there should be a *conscious decision* to eat or not to eat. In order to lose weight, I had to learn to be confident enough in my decision making to be proactive, rather than just reactive to the delicious taste of the food. I learned that whatever I eat has consequences. I found myself publicly exhibiting my private overindulgences as evidenced by my larger pant sizes.

No matter what kind of family or home life you've had, it's never too late to develop a positive sense of self-worth. It is important to find the positives in our lives that support our self-confidence. The most important component of your overall personality is who you are inside, regardless of the external issues surrounding you. Being overweight often undermines the positive image we want to have. But we have to persevere in the knowledge that *we are who we are,* no matter what our bodies look like. We must be prepared to accept ourselves as we are, and then we will be ready to move to the next level—to make the changes that will allow our self-confidence to grow. I experienced many setbacks on my weight-loss journey, but each time I learned valuable lessons about myself.

Why Lose Weight?

In order to lose weight, you must know why you want to lose weight. This is the second component of Success Principle #2. First you must figure out how you got here, and then you must figure out why you want to change.

I used to try to lose weight because I wanted to wear a certain outfit to a special event. I used to diet because I feared what others would say about me. Now I realize that I was succumbing to external influences. True goals, on the other hand, are formed in *our own minds*. We are the creators of our goals. Losing weight is not so much a physical task as a mental challenge. You use your mind to set and achieve goals. If you want to lose weight, you can do it for one reason and one reason only. That reason is you.

You must carve out time for yourself to reflect on the importance of what you are doing. At each stage you must think of the larger goal and focus your desire. You have to stop making excuses and start taking positive action. You and your goals must become a priority in your life. Even if you begin with baby steps, moving forward is much better than standing still. In my weight-loss journey, I had to change my eating habits little by little rather than attempt fad diets that promised immediate results.

Losing to Win

Athletes become Olympians by focusing on the future and putting off instant gratification for a larger goal. They cannot live in a comfort zone. They have to make choices compatible with their goals and be responsible for their own decisions. This is why they are uncommon. Finally, they have to persevere through both physical and mental discomforts. By losing common goals, they become winners.

Why is it so hard to be a winner? Because in order to be a winner, you also have to be a loser. You must be willing to lose your comfortable anonymity and become uncommon. You have to lose the easy answers and self-defeating rationalizations that keep you common. You have to give up old habits and step out of your comfort zone. You have to lose the self-indulgent excuses that keep you from trying your best. You have to lose the focus on the here and now in order to sacrifice for the future. For people who choose to remain common, all these things seem like too much to lose.

It took many failures before I realized that lasting weight loss is an uncommon goal. It's a common dream, but an uncommon goal. According to Bill Toomey, one of the key elements in athletics is the ability to be honest with yourself. The same is true in pursuing any goal. In losing and keeping off 100 pounds, I have achieved abilities beyond weight loss. I can now honestly assess my situation in many contexts. I have learned the meaning of setting and achieving long-term goals. I have learned not to sabotage my own efforts.

I had a lot of old attitudes and habits to discard along the way. I had a lot to lose before I could win. I hope that my experiences will help you to become uncommon, so that you, too, can lose to win in the best Olympic spirit.

— 3 —

Success Principle #3:
Build a Strong Foundation

— 3 —

Success Principle #3:
Build a Strong Foundation

"Whatever we plant in our subconscious mind and nourish with repetition and emotion will one day become a reality."

—Earl Nightingale

My journey of weight loss involved not just my body, but also my mind. Like an Olympic athlete striving to be the best at her game, you must discipline your mind and your emotions. You have to believe that change is possible. "Nothing can shake my self-confidence," said skier and Olympic gold medalist Jean-Claude Killy. "When you reach a certain level, you never experience the slightest anxiety. There's never the slightest apprehension." [1]

Mind over Body

My cousin Angie understood the power of a strong mind and the benefits of believing in herself. When she was just 21 years old, Angie was diagnosed with muscular dystrophy and told that she would be confined to a wheelchair for the rest of her life. She had recently become a registered nurse and was now being told that she would never walk again. She became dependent on others for so many things, from getting out of bed and getting dressed to bathing.

Although she qualified for disability benefits, Angie decided to work and managed to hold down a full-time job as a district director in charge of regional fundraising for the Muscular Dystrophy Association. Despite her physical limitations, she went to work five days a week. Angie taught me to go after what I want in life and often told me that her healthy mind was her most valuable possession.

And what a strong mind it was! When Angie started gaining a bit of weight, she decided to drop a few pounds. But how? Exercise wasn't an option for Angie. Instead, she controlled her portion sizes to take off the weight. Angie had an indomitable will to excel despite the limits that her disability imposed on her. She was truly an uncommon person. Angie taught me to be happy that I can move my body freely. And by her example, she reminded me to believe in myself.

Build Your Foundation

If you think of your body as a house, your mind is the foundation. Without a strong foundation, a house will fall apart. The same is true with your mind and body. Your mind is also your most powerful tool. It can enable you to move ahead and accomplish great things. It even has the power to preview the outcome of your goal before you accomplish it. This popular technique is called visualization, and it's useful for overcoming difficulties on the path to achieving your goals. In a sense, visualization is nothing more than having a plan for your future achievements, goals, and objectives.

Visualization has been extremely helpful for me as I lost and continue to maintain my weight. It is true that permanent weight loss revolves around portion control and moderate exercise, but staying vigilant and achieving your goal relies on feeding your mind a healthy diet of motivational messages. If you constantly tell yourself that you're weak and worthless, your foundation will crumble. If your mind is full of negativity and fear, how will you ever have the courage to take on self-improvement projects for your body? But by feeding your mind positive affirmations, you will help to ensure the long-term success of any endeavor.

Dealing with Painful Comments

All of my young adult life, people said that I had "such a pretty face." I wondered: What did that say about the rest of me? That I was ugly as sin? One particularly painful incident has stuck with me all these years.

While visiting my aunt, some of her friends stopped by with their son, whom I knew from previous visits. We were about the same age and got along well, but had no romantic interest in each other. Both of us were single twenty-somethings, and his mother thought it would be nice if we dated. She made a comment to that effect during this visit, and her husband had the nerve to say to me, "You have such a pretty face, but you are just too fat for my son."

If I had been thinner, would I have been considered a more suitable date or a better person? Those comments made me cry silent tears, and I felt so belittled for being so big. Physical beauty is too often conflated with personal worth in our society. I was tired of being made to feel like a second-class citizen for not being able to lose weight during that period of my life. Everywhere I turned I saw messages that to be overweight is to be "bad." Even the Church ranks gluttony as one of the Seven Deadly Sins. The perceived message is the same time and time again: "No fat chicks."

The rudeness of my aunt's friend shocked me and opened my eyes to how insensitive people can be. Even though I was hurt at the time, his comments have had a positive long-term effect on me. I eventually realized that I was letting other people's opinions intimidate me. It took years to learn this invaluable lesson: I had to be confident of my own worth in order to take charge of my life and my weight.

Letting Go of the Past

Once I started gaining weight, I found myself living in the past as a defense mechanism. During my twenties, if the subject of weight came up in a group of friends, I'd say things like, "I was twenty pounds thinner when I was in high school." I would even show people my "before" pictures of a thinner, younger me. It was easier to think about the past because my present weight was too painful. Facing the present and doing something about it takes true self-confidence.

We must have the confidence to realize that we are responsible for what we become—whether that's positive or negative. Sometimes we find it easier to pursue success in other areas of our lives, such as going back to school or going after a promotion. We have the self-confidence to put ourselves forward in many arenas, take responsibility, and go for our goals. But in the arena of weight loss, external pressures often intimidate us.

When I learned not to let others define me, I released the power of mind over matter and took full responsibility for my own weight problem. You're just wasting time and energy if you blame your weight on your circumstances, your past, or other people. Wouldn't it be great to blame someone else? Like your mom and her cooking, or your dad and his rule to "clean your plate!" Or your friends who always asked you to go out for pizza. We want to blame other people. It lets us off the hook! I have some advice that may sound harsh: get over it. Your parents did their best to raise you. Your friends may be eating junk food, but ultimately you must decide what you put into your mouth.

My mom used to tell me that a person doesn't gain weight because it's too sunny outside. She meant that being overweight isn't something that just happens. Yes, there are certain genetic factors we can't control. But to a large extent, we control our weight by the food we put into our mouths. It's time to stop making excuses and face yourself in the mirror. I used to ask my mom, "Does it look like I gained weight?" Her reply was characteristically short and to-the-point. "Fran, does the mirror lie?" Her words sound mean, but they were said with love. She was trying to teach me to take an honest look at myself. When I could finally do that, I stopped making excuses and started taking action. Let go of the past. The past doesn't have to equal the present. Even if you've struggled with losing weight before, that doesn't mean you have to continue to struggle.

Taking Control

To build your self-confidence and strengthen your mind, you must realize that your actions have resulted in your excess weight. You are responsible for yourself. Here's the good news: if you got yourself into this mess, you can get yourself out! When you accept that truth and understand that you are a valuable human being the way you are, then you can take the first steps toward a healthier and thinner you. You have to be ready, as my grandmother always said, "to shed blood for what you want to achieve in life." That's an extreme saying, but I like it for the passion that it conveys.

We must learn to let our minds control our actions. We have to think like that Olympic athlete. Remember, we must become uncommon in order to achieve permanent weight loss. As you progress on your own path, your confidence will increase. And one day, you'll realize that you no longer feel so apprehensive.

It's not whether you get knocked down. It's whether you get back up again.

~Vince Lombardi

We can do anything we want to if we stick to it long enough.

~Helen Keller

~ 4 ~

Success Principle #4:
Be Passionate

— 4 —

Success Principle #4:
Be Passionate

"I learned that the only way you are going to get anywhere in life is to work hard at it. Whether you're a musician, a writer, an athlete, or a businessman, there is no getting around it. If you do, you'll win—if you don't, you won't."
—Bruce Jenner, Decathlon Olympic Gold Medalist

Losing weight requires constant self-discipline and hard work. We've looked at how a strong mind can help you to reach your goal. But you must have both your head and your heart in the game. You can't be disciplined and work hard if you aren't motivated. Let's examine how I found my passion.

Getting Started

Sometimes it takes a traumatic event before we're ready to change. For me, it wasn't until I suffered a fall at work and had third-degree sprains to my ankle and arm that I realized I had to lose weight. I felt immeasurable embarrassment and humiliation as two people had to not only help me up but also transport me to the hospital. When I saw my emergency room X-rays, I noticed how small my bones were. I was amazed that such little bones were supporting so much flesh. The doctor said that both my ankle and arm were severely sprained and that I had to take it easy for a while. I was so transfixed on those X-rays that I barely heard a word he said. I decided then and there to take control of my life and free myself of my weight problem. I needed to develop a plan, and I needed to do it right away.

I knew I had to reclaim my life, but I had no idea how. I began reading about weight loss, metabolism, responsible choices, conscious decisions, muscular strength, cardiovascular endurance, abdominal fitness, heart disease, and the relationship between exercise and diseases. I read everything I could get my hands on. I learned to cook. Very slowly I started the habit of exercising. I followed the golden weight-loss rule: take in fewer calories and exercise more. I stopped wishing and dreaming and came up with a plan of action to summit my mountain, one small step at a time.

I took one of my first baby steps on a beautiful, sunny day in June after I recovered from the fall. I decided to go for a walk. My mom and our neighbor Jane had been begging me for years to walk with them. But at five feet one inch and 220 pounds, I never felt like exercising. So that day when I told my family I was going for a walk, they all looked at me in disbelief. I made it about a quarter of the way through the neighborhood that day, which equaled about one-fourth of a mile.

Another baby step was learning to cook. Before this, my idea of cooking dinner was calling for a pizza. But I made a commitment to myself to learn to cook healthy meals—and I did. I read a wide assortment of cookbooks and looked for simple recipes. I learned to read and understand food labels and did my best to stay away from unhealthy things like high fructose corn syrup and hydrogenated vegetable oils. It wasn't always easy, and I wasn't always happy about it. I often felt that I was limiting myself and making sacrifices by not allowing myself to eat whatever I wanted.

But those sacrifices were necessary to reclaim my life and my weight. Society loves the thin and healthy, but you have to stay focused in order to take the steps necessary to accomplish this goal. Your closest friends, family members, and colleagues may be puzzled by your new actions. Some of them may make negative comments. Stick with your determination. Eventually, most of them will turn into your best support system. And if they don't, they are the ones with the problem, not you. Stay the course. You must be ready to take them on, or even better—ignore them. If you can undergo this type of journey, your life will change forever in a positive way. Mine certainly did.

Passion Equals Motivation

How do you get and stay motivated? You need passion. Passion fuels motivation. Even though it would have been easy for my cousin Angie to give up and feel sorry for herself, she learned to live with passion. Despite being confined to a wheelchair, she stayed motivated. She often told me: "Without dreams and passion, life just becomes a list of boring things that we have to do."

Once you identify what has held you back in the past and then formulate a plan to turn your dreams into goals, what will keep you motivated to get fit, lose weight, and eat well? Passion is what will drive you to take care of yourself every day.

People often ask me how I have stayed motivated for so long. I care about myself passionately. I value who I am and want to honor that self-worth. And the more you work toward your goal, the more courage you'll have to keep going. We all face setbacks along the road to our goals. But if we keep moving forward, we'll acquire that momentum that helps us to forge ahead.

The greatest obstacle to passion is fear—oftentimes fear of the truth. The truth was that I was overweight and desperately needed to reclaim my life. But looking at the truth head-on can be frightening, because once we confront the truth, we can begin to change. That puts the responsibility squarely on our shoulders. And that can be scary!

I overcame this fear by using visualization and positive self-talk to promote mental toughness. I learned to reprogram my mind. There's no magic bullet for weight loss, even though there are dozens of diets and pills that promise to make you thin. Diets and supplements don't work. Making lifestyle changes is the only way to *change your life*.

Say No to Diets

Lasting weight loss seems like it should be simple: take in fewer calories, exercise more, and you'll maintain your ideal weight. If only it were as easy to do as to say! The disheartening statistic is that 99 percent of all people who lose weight on a diet gain it back again.[2, 3] For twelve years I allowed myself to be part of that "yo-yo diet" syndrome—weight loss followed by weight gain. I tried the grapefruit diet, the soup diet, the three-day quick fix, diet shakes, and others that I can't even remember. I was looking to external factors for my weight-loss answer.

After years of dieting, I realized that diets don't work. I don't even use the word "diet" anymore. To me, a diet is something you start and stop. This approach only works temporarily. Because they are temporary, diets just leave you frustrated by undermining your hard work. Diets indicate that certain foods are off-limits—*forever*. That's just not realistic. If you're going to be disciplined for the long-haul, you must have a plan that you can live with. When I was dieting, I hated the restrictions of "good" and "bad" foods. I finally decided that no food should be off-limits forever. My success came from controlling my portion sizes and exercising. I love ice cream, and I still eat it a few times a week. Why should I give it up forever if I don't gorge myself on it? I can have a scoop now and then.

You Have the Power

The real "secret" to achieving any goal lies in each one of us. As Glinda the Good Witch told Dorothy in *The Wizard of Oz*, "You always had the power." The real secret is a choice that I make consistently. I wake up each morning and decide if I will allow myself to slide back to 220 pounds or if I will choose to maintain my current weight. It's a choice I make over and over again every single day, all day long.

Stop Comparing Yourself

In order to be successful with your weight-loss journey, you have to stop comparing yourself to other people. We all know someone who seems to be able to eat and eat without ever gaining weight. So what? You don't know what he or she does in private. Maybe he exercises like a maniac seven days a week. Or maybe the only meal she's eaten all day is the one you see her eating. Besides, everyone's metabolism is different. You are not other people, so stop judging yourself by external standards. You are the only person you need to be concerned with. You know what you eat, how often you exercise, and what you need to do to be healthy. I'm not saying that any of this is easy, especially in the beginning. It's hard work. But you're worth it.

Overcoming Challenges

During the first six months of trying to lose weight, I often felt like Don Quixote de La Mancha tilting at windmills and following an impossible dream. But I persisted because I knew that it was up to me to determine if I would succeed or fail. Some of the people in my life weren't very supportive. They made negative comments that I could have let undermine my hard work. But I persevered. When they told me I would never lose so much weight, or that I would gain it all back, or that I was trying to do the impossible, I took those words as a challenge to work even harder. This was my quest. I would not allow other people's words to tear me down.

It's important to note that although I was in control of my journey, I wasn't alone. While I ignored the negativity around me, I welcomed encouragement from others, like my mother. My mom loves to walk and has always managed to carve out time for herself. She taught me that I need to exercise to see weight-loss results and encouraged me to start walking during those early months. The good thing about walking, she said, is that you don't need anything but a good pair of sneakers. There is no expensive gym to join or new skills to learn. She said, "Fran, you need to *move*. You don't need a personal trainer to be thin. It doesn't matter if you're rich or poor; we are all made equal by our hard work."

When I had 100 pounds to lose, I never thought about all the weight at once. I focused on ten pounds at a time. I did that ten times. It took me two full years to lose 100 pounds.

I achieved my goal in 1997, but there was another goal in front of me: maintaining the weight loss. Three years after reaching my goal weight, I faced a hurdle. I developed a planter's wart on the bottom of my right foot and neglected it for a summer. By September I was in a lot of pain and had to have the wart surgically removed. I couldn't walk with a normal stride for three months, but I would wrap my foot to exercise. This aggravated the wound and my doctor told me to stop working out for a week.

I allowed one week to turn into three months and gained twelve pounds. Those twelve pounds led to another thirteen. Before I knew it I had gained back a quarter of the weight I'd lost. I was devastated. I carried around those twenty-five extra pounds for two more years. In June 2004, I recommitted to reaching my goal weight and took off the twenty-five pounds, again by portion control and moderate exercise. This time it took me a full six months to achieve my goal. Since then I have continued to maintain my height-appropriate weight.

The challenges, setbacks, and successes of my weight-loss journey have taught me that permanent weight loss is possible. As the saying goes, if you can believe it, you can do it. You must stay the course and persevere. If you stumble and fall, you must get back up and keep going in the direction of your goal. No one else will do it for you. It's your commitment and passion that will help you to win the race.

Many of life's failures are people who had not realized how close they were to success when they gave up.

~Thomas Edison

Being defeated is often a temporary condition. Giving up is what makes it permanent.

~Marilyn Vos Savant

— 5 —

Success Principle #5:
Never Give Up

— 5 —

Success Principle #5:
Never Give Up

"Our greatest weakness lies in giving up. The most certain way to succeed is to always try just one more time."

—*Thomas Edison*

Even though I achieved my desired weight and have maintained it for over twelve years, I must recommit to my goals every single day. That said, I don't look at maintenance as a constant struggle anymore. It's become part of my life, part of who I am, and part of the way I make decisions.

But it doesn't always happen automatically. Some days are harder than others. When I feel discouraged, I get out my size 22 pants, hold them next to me while looking in the mirror, and remind myself of what I really enjoy: *I enjoy feeling healthy*. I didn't realize how bad I felt until I began to lose weight and started to feel better. By keeping that good feeling in focus, I recommit to maintaining my weight every single day.

I even enjoy exercising now. In fact, exercising is the easy part for me. That's my time that I have carved out for myself. It's so much easier and more enjoyable to replace your worn-out sneakers than to have quadruple bypass surgery. I know that a lot of people, maybe most, don't share my love of exercise. If that's the case for you, try thinking of exercise as a means to an end. It's just a way to be healthier and feel better. We routinely do other tasks that we may not enjoy, like paying the bills or doing laundry. But these are necessary parts of life. They keep us from wrecking our financial credit or having to wear dirty underwear. We may not love the act of doing those things, but we enjoy the results. It's the same with exercise.

Exercise does more than keep my body healthy. "To exercise at or near capacity is the best way I know of reaching a true introspective state. If you do it right, it can open all kinds of inner doors," said Al Oerter, a four-time Olympic discus gold medalist. One of these "inner doors" is a deep sense of enjoyment.

Take my friend Bill as an example. Due to an unfortunate farming accident, Bill had his leg amputated below the knee. Despite this, Bill still makes time to exercise on an elliptical machine. He says that he exercises because it makes him feel good inside and out. Like Bill, I feel better when I exercise. I truly enjoy the new and different challenges I encounter every time I change my routine.

But I remember what it felt like when walking for just a few blocks was so difficult for me. That memory is another way that I motivate myself to continue to live a healthy lifestyle. I don't want to have to start that journey all over again.

We live in a society filled with instant gratification. Weight loss doesn't work that way. I can't say this enough: there is no magic formula. You must be willing to put in the time to lose weight in a healthy and lasting manner. It can be a long journey, but it is so worthwhile. I am a living example that change is possible. Are you ready to do what it takes? Are you ready to commit to this journey?

Dealing with Setbacks

Along the way, you will experience setbacks. This is a normal part of trying to reach a goal, and can feel especially true with weight loss. Your weight-loss efforts will plateau many times. You have to be patient. I once went into a weight plateau for twelve weeks, but I never gave up.

Expect to feel a little bit sore from exercising, especially in the beginning. Expect some people to misunderstand or be unsupportive of your efforts. This doesn't mean that you should give up. Yes, even the most well-designed plan can be sabotaged, but *not* by negative comments from close friends, colleagues, and family members. Only you can sabotage it. This means that you have the responsibility of safeguarding your efforts and attitude.

But sometimes setbacks come from within us. If I have a day when I eat too much or make unhealthy food choices, I don't beat myself up about it. I remind myself that tomorrow is another day and recommit to my goal. If you have a bad day, do your best to get back on track so that one day doesn't turn into two or three. Also, don't be consumed with time and how long it's taking you to lose weight. Experts agree that losing one to two pounds of weight a week is a healthy way to do it. It may not seem like a lot at first, but results come with consistency. I have seen big results over a long period of time.

Celebrating Achievement

As you work toward your weight-loss goals and strive to maintain your success, it's important to celebrate your achievements. In fact, it's a necessary component when you're in the middle of a pound-by-pound fight. Don't forget to congratulate yourself for your hard work. Surround yourself with people who will support you and celebrate with you. Don't let the negative comments of naysayers distract you from your goals or diminish the pride you take in your efforts. As I struggled with my own weaknesses during my weight-loss journey, I have become more forgiving of others' weaknesses. I have found the ability to enjoy other people with all their foibles and to enjoy my own company too. The bottom line is to be kind to yourself and to others, even if they're not kind to you. It might not help you to lose more weight, but it's good karma.

Finding Inspiration

As you build your support system, look for inspiration from the uncommon people around you. One of the people who inspired me was my high school friend Dawn. Although she was only in my life for a short time, the lessons she taught me are priceless.

Dawn was diagnosed with an aggressive form of diabetes when she was just nine months old. As a result, she had to be extremely careful about everything she ate. Despite her vigilance, Dawn developed serious complications from diabetes in her twenties. She endured retinopathy, kidney failure, and amputations before her death at age 36.

Her ordeal influenced me from a young age not to take my body for granted. So many people pollute their bodies with alcohol, drugs, and too much bad food—all by choice. Through no fault of her own, Dawn dealt with juvenile diabetes and a body that failed her. But she watched me go through my weight-loss journey and was very happy for me. Her support along the way was invaluable.

"Learn from me," Dawn said. "My body is wearing out and soon it won't be able to take much more. If you do nothing else in your life, protect your cardiovascular system. I won't always be here to support you, but don't ever be afraid to get older, because it is an honor and a privilege to get older. I am not going to earn that privilege, but you are. So take care of yourself." Dawn knew that good health is a gift. She taught me that we need to safeguard this gift. Don't let your fear of failing or your desire to stay in your comfort zone keep you from making the most of the one life you've been given. No matter how old you are, or how much weight you have to lose, or what shape your body is in, you can decide each day to make healthy choices and work toward a better you. It's never too late to start or to recommit.

Don't Just "Try"

At some tough places along my weight-loss journey, people told me, "It looks like you're losing weight." I tended to downplay it and say, "I'm trying." But I realize that I wasn't just *trying*; I was actually *doing* it. Looking back, I think this word choice could have sabotaged my own efforts. The idea of "trying" can become an easy out; a way of avoiding real success. By saying "I'm trying," there was a little bit of doubt in my mind. *"Am I just trying or am I actually doing it?"* I would think. Trying is just the first step. You have to risk everything and get beyond trying to a real commitment in order to reach real achievement. You have to risk the failures to enjoy the successes. Whether you lose nine pounds or ninety, it's not an easy feat. Be proud of your efforts and know that good results will follow your hard work.

Conclusion

I once heard a sermon in which the priest asked us to imagine living in a world without the possibility of change. How depressing and overwhelming that would be! But thankfully, he pointed out, we know that change is possible. Yet we often feel that *others* should change, or that *circumstances* should be different. Self-righteousness knows no culpability.

Nonetheless, we also know that the only thing we can change is *ourselves*. If we want change to happen, we must be the ones to change.

You must have a deep belief that you can change and that permanent weight loss is possible. You don't have to be stuck at your current weight. Too often, people who desire to achieve permanent weight loss can't imagine themselves in a different way. Once we can envision the possibility for change, we can change our desires into achievable goals. For this we need uncommon vision. Fear subverts our goals—fear of change, fear of discomfort, but most of all, fear of failure. To overcome these fears, we need uncommon courage. To get from a goal to an achievement, we need understanding of ourselves, self-confidence in our abilities, and passion to keep going.

Sometimes people ask me if I'm angry that I allowed myself to be so overweight for so long. I don't have a ready answer for that question. But here's what I do know: being overweight and then losing the weight and keeping it off has made me who I am. The experience has taught me three valuable lessons in life: how to cope with frustration, how to celebrate the inner beauty of myself and others, and most importantly, how to be forgiving of weaknesses—my own and those of other people.

I believe in the Golden Rule: "Love your neighbor as yourself." I realized that to follow it, I had to love myself first. I also came to understand that uncovering or developing a strong sense of self-worth is paramount to making lasting changes. Only then could I declare the independence of my psyche. The biggest loss is that of independence, and loving food more than self is synonymous with that loss. Food used to control me, but there has been a shift in power. I no longer cede power to food. I have declared my independence from this dependence.

The very first step in achieving permanent weight loss is to honestly look at your life and decide if you are ready to begin the journey. I knew I was ready for the journey in June of 1995 because for the first time, I could admit to myself that it was time to step out of my comfort zone and lose the security that it had provided for so many years. I stopped looking for a quick fix and stopped making excuses. I know that you can do the same!

Opportunity is missed by most people because it is dressed in overalls and looks like work.

~Thomas Edison

Practical Success Tips

Practical Success Tips

As I stated at the beginning, this is not a how-to book. Just like every person is different, every person will have a different weight-loss journey. So far, I've focused on the success principles that form the foundation for achieving and maintaining a weight-loss goal. But because so many people ask me for my "secret," I'll share some of my practical tips.

Remember, there is no secret! There is no magic formula. Learn all you can about good nutrition and exercise, and then devise a plan that works for your body, your mind, and your spirit. Here's what worked for me.

Food and Cooking

I often hear people complain that it is difficult to cook for one person. I disagree. I know that I am no competition for those celebrity TV chefs, but I regularly cook for myself. I taught myself to cook and stick to it by choosing very simple recipes that are big on flavor and low on calories.

I said there is no secret to permanent weight loss, but here's an invaluable tip: get organized with your food. You must plan your meals ahead of time and be prepared to cook. Because of my hectic schedule, I usually cook a week's worth of meals on the weekend. I cook a couple of different items, usually on a Sunday, and this is my lunch and dinner for the entire week. As a bonus, I estimate that I save about $750 a year by packing a lunch instead of eating out. What to pack is usually a no-brainer: I just use the leftovers from the last night's dinner. So although I'm cooking for one, I can cook enough for several meals. (See the Appendix for some of my favorite recipes.)

Beyond the mental preparation and commitment that we've explored so far, there are two main parts to weight loss: eating and exercising. You must control what goes into your body and what effort you exert. Don't be fooled into thinking that exercising allows you to eat any amount of whatever you want. In addition to choosing healthy, nutritious foods, make sure that you control your portion size. Take the time to learn about good nutrition and appropriate serving sizes. Educating yourself is one of the best things you can do. Remember, losing weight is largely a mental process. Your mind is a powerful tool.

Off-limit Foods

Should you avoid dairy? Meat? Carbs? I eat them all. No food is off-limits for me. Of course, anything in excess can be bad. But most of us need the right balance of protein, carbohydrates, and healthy fats even when we're working to lose weight. With the exception of dietary restrictions and health conditions, the total elimination of any one food category could set you up for failure. I already went down that road.

What happens if you declare all pizza or cookies or ice cream off-limits, forever and ever? You instantly want to eat mounds of that forbidden food! But if you know that you can have a sensible portion of these delights every so often, you can keep yourself in check.

Even the best designed plan will not work if you constantly feel deprived or let yourself get bored with your food. I have never given up what I enjoy eating. I just make healthier choices. For example, I love baked potatoes. Now, instead of having one loaded with butter, bacon, and sour cream, I just eat a better baked potato. I might put a little bit of butter on it for flavor or maybe use some salsa. I also love ice cream, and I don't have to give it up. Sometimes I'll have a decadent frozen custard, but sometimes I'll substitute a yummy frozen yogurt with sprinkles instead. I now view myself as an active person who makes good food choices most of the time. But I'm never going to be perfect. That is just not realistic. So I allow myself to have a treat from time to time.

Eating with Friends

When I was overweight, I never watched what I ate, especially on special occasions like dinner out with friends or while on vacation. But that has changed. Just because you are on vacation or eating out doesn't mean that you have to abandon your daily routine. The same rules apply at all times. If a restaurant serves a super-size portion, I either share the entrée with a friend or take half home with me. I don't panic when I go out or on vacation. I just allow that time to be an extension of my everyday life. I'll eat dessert on vacation, but not every day. Even if I don't make it to the gym for my normal workout while I'm away from home, I make sure that I stay active.

While vacationing in California recently, I discovered Sprinkles Cupcakes in Beverly Hills. These small cakes pack a big wallop. They appealed to me on so many levels: they're beautiful to look at, tasty to eat, and don't contain any trans fat. Did I enjoy a few cupcakes while I was there? You bet I did!

But back when I was on the diet roller coaster, desserts were off-limits, which made them all the more desirable because of their scarcity. I wouldn't give myself permission to taste even a bite of a cupcake without feeling guilty back then. I ceded power to the cupcake, instead of being in charge of my own feelings and behaviors. Looking back, I realize that what made me crave those desserts in the first place was this total deprivation. By not allowing myself to enjoy any sweet morsel, I put extra value on the sweets.

But now that I'm in control of my actions and understand the value of making conscious decisions, I allow my life to be sprinkled with all sorts of good things. To go through life saying that you'll never taste another piece of birthday cake ever again is only going to set you up for sabotaging your weight loss. It's important to remember our focus: not the perfect diet plan, but continuous healthy habits. I have slowly taught myself to eat desserts—like everything else—in moderation.

I have learned to make big changes in my life by making small changes with food and exercise. I no longer feel compelled to act based on my circumstances. I don't have to eat what everyone else is eating. Enjoying the company of friends does not mean eating heavy foods or overeating. Besides, conversation is easier if your mouth isn't constantly full!

Choose Your Path

Weight loss is very person-specific. I can't tell you what you need to eat. You must chart your own course by sifting through the information and deciding what is appropriate for you. This could take the form of a sensible weight-loss program, many of which are commercially available, or you may design your own. You may want to buy other books that deal with healthy eating or exercise. It is also advisable that you discuss your diet plan with a medical professional. Whatever you decide to do, you must choose a path that allows you to make mistakes and then get back on track. The weight-loss program you choose is just the vehicle to your dream. And the dream is to reclaim your life. Losing weight just doesn't happen—*you make it happen.*

Choose Your Journey

These five success principles can motivate you to choose other difficult journeys beyond weight loss. Pursuing such quests allows you to be more self-reliant and gain more wisdom. You will become more aware of what you can and can't control, what you can change, and what you must accept with good grace. The first step of any journey can be a difficult choice, but taking it will lead you on a quest that will change you into a new person.

5 Success Principles

1. Change desires into goals.
   Stop wishing.
   Start doing.

2. Identify how you got here.
   Look back to see where you came from.
   Choose where you will be going next.

3. Build a strong foundation.
   Do your homework.
   Become informed.

4. Be passionate.
   Praise yourself.
   Rejoice in small successes.

5. Never give up.
   Follow the path you've laid out.
   Choose the long term over the short term.

Appendix: Recipes

Appendix: Recipes

Poor eating habits used to weigh me down. My zest for life rose as my weight dropped. As I learned to take a closer look within, I rediscovered the happy person that I truly am. But that happy self had become a slave to bad eating habits and no exercise. Today, the prisoner within has been liberated. Learning how to cook and take care of myself was a major component in obtaining my freedom.

Included here are thirty of my favorite recipes, some invented and others gleaned from here and there, but rewritten to suit my nutritional needs and my taste buds. I challenge you to create one new dish each day of the month, and I hope each one encourages you to continue cooking tasty, healthy, and hearty meals!

Lighter Meals

Rustic Bean Soup with Garlic

Delicious flavor. Add a salad and crusty bread for a complete meal.

Ingredients:
1 1/2 tablespoons olive oil
1 large carrot, diced
1 cup onion, chopped
4 large garlic cloves, minced
3 cups escarole cut into small pieces
3–4 cups reduced-sodium chicken broth
2 (15 oz.) cans white kidney beans, rinsed
1 large can (16–20 oz.) no-salt-added diced
tomatoes, drained
2 dried bay leaves
1/2 teaspoon ground sage
1/2 teaspoon basil
2 tablespoons Parmesan cheese
Flavored croutons as desired

Put oil in a large, heavy pot and heat to medium-low. Add the next three ingredients. Sauté until onions are translucent, about 7 minutes. Add escarole and cook for 3 minutes, stirring occasionally. Add broth, beans, tomatoes, bay leaves, sage, and basil. Bring to a boil. Reduce heat, cover, and simmer until escarole is tender, about 20 to 25 minutes. Season to taste. Remove bay leaves. Serve with Parmesan cheese and/or croutons.

Tri-colored Pepper Soup

Comfort food in a bowl

Ingredients:
1/2 pound ground turkey breast
1 teaspoon olive oil
1/2 cup yellow bell pepper, chopped
1/2 cup red bell pepper, chopped
1 cup green bell pepper, chopped
1 cup onion, chopped
1/4 teaspoon black pepper
1 (14 oz.) can reduced-sodium chicken broth
1 (10 oz.) can RO*TEL Original Diced Tomatoes and Green Chilies, undrained (usually found in the international section of the grocery store)
1 (10 3/4 oz.) can low-fat, low-salt tomato soup, undiluted
1/2 tablespoon worcestershire sauce
1/2 teaspoon garlic powder
1 1/2 cups hot cooked brown rice

Heat oil in a small Dutch oven to medium-high heat. Add chopped peppers and onion and cook 5 minutes. Add turkey and cook about 10 minutes or until meat is browned, stirring to crumble. Vegetables should be tender and meat cooked through. Add chicken broth, RO*TEL, and tomato soup. Add worcestershire sauce and garlic powder. Season to taste with pepper. Bring to a boil. Reduce heat and simmer 45 minutes. Meanwhile, cook rice according to package directions. Add the cooked rice to soup during the last 10 minutes of cooking.

Nancy's Frittata
Breakfast, lunch, or dinner . . . perfect anytime

Ingredients:
3 tablespoons olive oil
1/2 cup sweet onion, chopped
1 medium yellow banana pepper, chopped
3 cups zucchini, chopped
2 eggs, beaten
Freshly ground black pepper, to taste
1 teaspoon dried oregano
Sea salt, to taste

In cast-iron skillet, heat oil to medium-high. Add onion and banana pepper; sauté 3 to 5 minutes. Add zucchini, cover skillet, and reduce heat to medium-low. Cook for 12 minutes or until zucchini is tender. Uncover and add beaten eggs to skillet, stirring constantly until eggs are cooked.

Serving suggestions:

Breakfast: Serve with fresh fruit salad and orange juice
Lunch: Serve with Tuscini Soup and crusty bread
Dinner: Serve with Turkey Press sandwich

Barb's Garden Scramble
Veggie lover's delight

Ingredients:
3 tablespoons canola oil
1 cup sliced zucchini or other squash
1 cup each broccoli spears, green beans, chopped celery, onion rounds, and cut sweet red or yellow pepper
2 tomatoes, chopped or 1 lb. can stewed tomatoes
Fresh basil and/or other Italian seasonings
Sliced provolone, optional

Heat oil. Stir fry zucchini, broccoli, beans, celery, onions, and peppers for about 20 minutes. The peppers need the least cooking and are even good a bit crunchy, so add them last. Add fresh tomatoes or canned tomatoes along with your favorite Italian seasonings. Stir. Top each serving with a slice of provolone or your favorite cheese (can be added in the skillet if all the dish will be eaten). Serves 4 to 6.

Barb's Rhubarb Sauce
Partner in Paradise

Ingredients:
Approximately 4 cups rhubarb
1/2 cup water
1 lb. canned fruit of your choice or fresh fruit
1/4 cup sugar (omit if using canned fruit)

Chop up four long stacks of rhubarb and cook in water with sugar. If using canned fruit, cook the rhubarb in the drained fruit juice. Rhubarb will make its own juice. Take off the burner and add the drained fruit or fresh fruit. Cool. The rhubarb will partner with any fruit, including pineapple, mandarin oranges, strawberries, papaya, guava, apples, or pears.

Serving suggestions: Tastes excellent with pineapple served over a pork or ham dish. Eat hot as is or serve warm over vanilla ice cream. Makes a great substitute for jam on your toast.

Tuscini Soup
A taste of the Mediterranean

Ingredients:
4 cups chopped zucchini
1 1/2 cups chopped potatoes
1 tablespoon chopped banana pepper, or to taste
1/2 cup chopped sweet onion
2 (14.5 oz.) cans low-salt stewed tomatoes
1 large clove garlic, chopped
Olive oil
Chicken stock

Add olive oil to Dutch oven to coat bottom of pan. Heat pan to medium-high. Add garlic, onion, and banana pepper; sauté. Add potatoes, tomatoes, and chicken stock to cover potatoes. Bring to high simmer, reduce heat, and cover, cooking for 20 minutes. Remove lid from pot, stir, and add zucchini. Continue cooking 5 minutes, adding chicken stock if needed.

Turkey Press
A sandwich with attitude

Ingredients:
2 slices of whole grain bread
2–3 slices of oven-roasted turkey breast
3–4 rehydrated sundried tomatoes
Fresh mozzarella cheese
Pesto sauce

Preheat countertop grill or panini press. Arrange sandwich by layering turkey, tomatoes, and cheese on bread which has been spread with 1 tablespoon of pesto sauce. Place sandwich on grill and press tightly for 3 to 4 minutes. Serve with pickle spear and fresh fruit.

Gyro Burger

An authentic Greek sandwich served with fresh toppings and a creamy dressing

Dressing:
1 cup plain, nonfat yogurt
1/4 teaspoon dill weed
1/4 teaspoon sea salt
1 garlic clove, minced
1 tablespoon fresh lemon juice

Burger:
1/2 pound ground turkey
1/2 pound lean ground lamb
1/2 teaspoon sea salt
1/4 teaspoon Mrs. Dash seasoning
1 garlic clove, minced

Toppings:
1 medium onion, sliced
1 large ripe tomato, sliced
Romaine lettuce, chopped

4–6 whole wheat flatbreads

Dressing: Combine ingredients and chill.

Burger: Combine all ingredients. Mix well. Shape into 4 to 6 patties. Grill or pan fry patties until cooked through. (I do this on a countertop grill.)

Assembly: Put one patty near edge of the flatbread. Place desired toppings on burger; drizzle with dressing. Fold ends of flatbread together and enjoy.

Greek Garden Salad
Crisp greens tastefully dressed

Salad:
1 bunch romaine
2 medium tomatoes, chopped
2 cucumbers, peeled and sliced
1 red onion, sliced
1/2 cup Greek olives
Feta cheese

Dressing:
1/2 cup fresh lemon juice
1/4 cup olive oil
1/2 teaspoon sea salt (optional)
Freshly ground pepper
2 cloves minced garlic
2 teaspoons dried oregano

Rough chop lettuce and place into salad bowl. Layer tomato and cucumber slices over lettuce. Top with onions and olives. Combine ingredients for the dressing (can be made ahead). Drizzle over the salad and sprinkle with feta.

Roasted Red Pepper Dip
Smooth, satisfying, and full of flavor

Ingredients:
3 cloves of roasted garlic, mashed
2 tablespoons olive oil
1 tablespoon balsamic vinegar
1 (15 oz.) can garbanzo beans, drained
1 (12 oz.) jar roasted red peppers, drained
1/8 teaspoon sea salt
1 tablespoon cilantro, chopped

Whisk together the garlic, olive oil, balsamic vinegar, salt, and cilantro. Puree the garbanzo beans and the red peppers in food processor while drizzling olive oil mixture into bean and pepper mixture. Pulse until smooth.

Serving suggestions:

Chill in a hollowed-out red pepper. Wonderful with toasted baguette slices.

Big G's Broccoli and Whole Wheat Pasta

A taste from the old country

Ingredients:
1/4 cup olive oil
2–3 garlic cloves, chopped
1 teaspoon red pepper flakes
1/4–1/2 pound whole wheat pasta (cook, drain, and keep warm)
Salt, to taste
Black pepper, to taste
Small head fresh broccoli (rinsed, drained, and cut into florets)

Heat oil in skillet over medium heat. Add garlic, flowerets, red pepper flakes, salt, and pepper. Sauté 3 to 4 minutes. Do not overcook broccoli. Pour mixture over hot pasta and toss. Sprinkle with grated Parmesan cheese if desired.

Oven-roasted Vegetables
Easy cooking technique, great results

Ingredients:
Butternut squash (already cubed from store)
Sweet potatoes, peeled and sliced
Broccoli florets, chopped
Fresh green beans
Carrots, peeled and sliced
Potatoes, peeled and sliced
Purple onion, peeled and sliced
Cold pressed olive oil
Sea salt and black pepper, to taste

Preheat oven to 400°. Rinse, cut, and chop vegetables. Place a single layer of vegetables on a cookie sheet. Drizzle vegetables with olive oil. Sprinkle with sea salt and black pepper. Roast vegetables until lightly brown, approximately 40 to 45 minutes, turning occasionally.

Oven-roasted Asparagus
Your taste buds will beg for more!

Ingredients:
Asparagus
Olive oil
Sea salt and black pepper, to taste

Preheat oven to 400°. Rinse and trim ends of asparagus. Place a single layer of asparagus on a cookie sheet and drizzle with cold pressed olive oil. Sprinkle with sea salt and black pepper. Roast until lightly brown, approximately 20 minutes. Turn once after the first 10 minutes.

Beans and Greens
Full of texture and great nutrition

Ingredients:
1 (6 oz.) bag baby spinach
1 (15.5 oz.) can white kidney beans
2–3 garlic cloves, chopped
Salt, to taste
Pepper, to taste
Olive oil, to taste

Wash spinach. Blanch the spinach in boiling water for approximately 30 seconds. Drain and put in serving bowl. Add rinsed and drained kidney beans. Add garlic, salt, pepper, and olive oil. Toss to combine.

Entrées

Fiesta Balsamic Glazed Chicken

Chicken never had it so good!

Ingredients:
1 teaspoon olive oil
5 garlic cloves, sliced
1 cup coarsely chopped sweet onion
4 boneless, skinless chicken breasts (medium-thin)
1/4 cup sliced red bell pepper
1/4 cup sliced green bell pepper
1/4 cup sliced yellow bell pepper
1/4 cup sliced orange bell pepper
(You can use all red, green, yellow, or all orange peppers. The mix simply adds more color to the dish.)
2 small celery stocks, diced
1 cup zucchini, diced
1/2 cup balsamic vinegar
1 teaspoon Mrs. Dash seasoning
1 (14–16 oz.) can no-salt-added diced tomatoes, undrained

Spray a large skillet with cooking spray and then heat the oil over medium-high heat. Add onions, bell peppers, celery, and garlic. Sauté for approximately 3 minutes. Add chicken; sauté about 4 minutes on each side or until lightly browned. Add balsamic vinegar, Mrs. Dash seasoning, and tomatoes. Reduce heat to medium-low and cook for about 20 minutes or until chicken is cooked through. Add zucchini during the last 10 minutes.

Fresh Veggie Fettuccine
A healthy classic

Ingredients:
1 tablespoon olive oil
1 small to medium onion, chopped
1/2 cup chopped red bell pepper
1/2 cup chopped green bell pepper
1/2 cup chopped yellow bell pepper
1/2 cup chopped zucchini
2 cups broccoli florets
1/2 cup evaporated skimmed milk
1 teaspoon fresh or dried basil
1/4 teaspoon black pepper
1 tomato, skinned and coarsely chopped
4 cups hot cooked whole wheat fettuccine noodles
1/2 cup grated Parmesan cheese

Heat oil in a nonstick skillet. Add bell peppers and sauté, stirring as needed, until onion is translucent, about 5 to 6 minutes. Add zucchini, broccoli, milk, basil, and black pepper; cover and cook until broccoli is tender-crisp, about 3 minutes. Add tomato and cook until heated through, about 1 minute. Meanwhile, cook fettuccine as directed on package. Place fettuccine in a medium serving bowl. Top with vegetable sauce mixture; toss to coat. Add cheese as desired.

Twice As Nice Chicken
*A simple sauté featuring two fabulous sauces**

Ingredients:
1 1/2 tablespoons butter
4 boneless thin chicken breasts
3 tablespoons flour
1 cup fat-free, reduced-sodium chicken broth
1/2 cup skim milk
2 tablespoons parsley
Cooking spray

*For dijon recipe, add 2 tablespoons country-style
  dijon mustard
*For pesto recipe, add 2 tablespoons prepared pesto

Spray skillet with cooking spray and melt butter
over medium heat. Add chicken breasts and sauté
about 5 minutes per side, or until lightly browned.
(To avoid dryness, do not overcook.) Remove
chicken. For the sauce, stir flour into pan drippings
and cook for 1 minute. Add the chicken broth and

milk, stirring constantly to avoid lumps, and cook until the sauce thickens and bubbles. Stir in pesto or mustard. Return the chicken to the skillet. Cover and cook over low heat for 10 minutes, or until chicken is cooked through. Sprinkle with parsley.

Sesame Chicken
Tender chicken stir-fry—delicious!

Ingredients:
1 pound (pre-cooking weight) boneless white meat chicken, cubed
2–4 cloves garlic, minced
1 tablespoon canola oil
1/2 red pepper, thinly sliced
1/2 yellow pepper, thinly sliced
1/2 green pepper, thinly sliced
1/2 orange pepper, thinly sliced
2 cups raw broccoli, thinly sliced
2 carrots, thinly sliced
4–6 green onions, thinly sliced
3 tablespoons cornstarch
1 1/2 cups chicken broth
1/3 cup low-sodium soy sauce
1/4 cup brown sugar
1/4 teaspoon cayenne pepper
1/4 teaspoon crushed hot pepper flakes, to taste
2 teaspoons sesame seeds, or to taste
Cooking spray

Heat a large, deep skillet over medium heat. Coat skillet with cooking spray. Heat oil in skillet; sauté chicken and garlic for 2 to 3 minutes, stirring frequently. Add red, yellow, green, and orange peppers, broccoli, and carrots to skillet and sauté for about 5 minutes, or until vegetables are crispy-tender and chicken is cooked through. Add half the onions about halfway through the sautéing process. Mix together cornstarch, chicken broth, soy sauce, brown sugar, and cayenne pepper. In a separate bowl, add cornstarch mixture and cook 2 minutes or until sauce thickens. Season to taste with hot pepper flakes and sesame seeds.

Serving suggestions:

For more fiber and a heartier taste, serve with brown rice cooked according to package directions.

Roasted Roughy
A seafood lover's delight

Ingredients:
4 (6 oz.) orange roughy fillets
1 (10 oz.) package frozen spinach, thawed
2 egg whites
3/4 cup whole wheat bread crumbs
4 teaspoons freshly grated Parmesan cheese
Cooking spray

Preheat oven to 400°. Place fish into shallow dish that has been lightly coated with cooking spray. In a small bowl, combine well-drained spinach, egg whites, whole wheat bread crumbs, and cheese. Mix until blended. Divide mixture evenly into 4 portions and place on fish. Sprinkle lightly with additional cheese and sweet red paprika. Bake for approximately 20 minutes.

Racz Fish
Fantastic fillet of sole

Ingredients:
1 lb. fillet of sole
2 tomatoes, thinly sliced
1 medium onion, thinly sliced
1 green pepper, thinly sliced
Sea salt, to taste
Pepper, to taste
Olive oil

Place fish into a shallow baking dish. Place tomatoes, onion, and pepper on fish. Drizzle with olive oil and bake at 350° for 15 to 20 minutes until fish flakes. Remove from oven and add sea salt and pepper to taste.

Italian Stuffed Squash
Pleases both the eyes and taste buds!

Ingredients:
4 medium yellow squash
4 ounces loose Italian sausage (sweet or hot)
1 medium onion, chopped
1/2 green pepper, chopped
1/2 red pepper, chopped
2–3 slices dried Italian bread, crumbled
Salt and pepper, to taste
Parmesan cheese, to taste

In a large skillet, sauté peppers, onions, and sausage over medium heat. Crumble sausage until thoroughly cooked. Pour off excess fat. Meanwhile, cook squash in boiling water until soft. Cut lengthwise and scoop out pulp. Place pulp into mixing bowl and add bread crumbs, seasoning, and sausage; mix. (To hold mixture together, add water.) Place mixture into squash shells, then transfer to a cookie sheet. Bake at 375° until brown. Top with cheese.

Desserts

Tropical Smoothie
A taste of the islands

Ingredients:
1 (8 oz.) container plain yogurt
1/4 cup lime juice
1/4 cup pineapple juice
3 tablespoons honey
1 1/2 cups frozen pineapple chunks
1 1/2 cups frozen banana slices
1 cup cubed or crushed ice

Place all ingredients in blender in the order listed. Blend until smooth.

Tip: Try your own favorite combinations. For variations of your own favorite flavors, chop and peel desired fruit into small chunks. Freeze fruit into individual portions. Use as directed per recipe procedure.

Razzmatazz
Power yourself healthy

Ingredients:
1/2 cup raspberries or blueberries (or your own favorite berry combinations)
3 oz. French vanilla yogurt
1/2 cup pomegranate juice

Place all ingredients in blender in the order listed.
Blend until smooth.

Triple Berry Smoothie
Goodness in a glass

Ingredients:
1 cup ice cubes or crushed ice
1 cup almond milk
1 frozen peeled banana
1 cup mixed frozen berries (raspberries, blueberries, blackberries)
1 tablespoon almond butter or peanut butter

Place the ice cubes into a blender and crush until you have a snow cone–like base. Then, place remaining ingredients in blender in the order listed. Blend until consistency is thick but smooth. Yields two servings. Tip: Try your own favorite flavor combinations.

Marathon Muffins
Your sweet tooth will thank you.

Ingredients:
1 (15 oz.) can plain pumpkin*
1 box chocolate cake mix
1/4 teaspoon cinnamon
Powdered sugar (optional)

Preheat oven to 350º. Combine canned pumpkin, cinnamon, and cake mix. Mixture will be thick. Place paper liners into 12-count muffin tin. Pour batter into liners evenly. Bake at 350º for 20 to 23 minutes. Sprinkle each muffin lightly with powdered sugar when cooled, if desired.

*1 cup applesauce mixed with 1/2 cup mashed banana can be substituted for the pumpkin.

Almond Biscotti

Light and crunchy. Perfect for dunking. (See Choffee recipe)

Ingredients:
1 cup unsalted butter, softened
2 1/2 cups sugar (set 1/2 cup aside)
6 eggs
2 teaspoons vanilla
4 cups all-purpose flour
4 teaspoons baking powder
Pinch of salt
1 cup sliced natural almonds
4 teaspoons milk

Preheat oven to 375°. Cream butter and 2 cups sugar. Add eggs one at a time. Beat well after each addition (batter should be a light yellow). Stir in vanilla. In a separate bowl, combine dry ingredients. Fold into creamed mixture. Stir in almonds. Line baking sheets with parchment paper. Divide dough into fourths; spread into four 12-inch-by-3-inch rectangles on parchment paper. Brush with milk and sprinkle with remaining sugar. Bake at 375° for 15 to 20 minutes until golden brown and firm to the touch. Remove the rectangles and place them on wire racks to cool for 15 minutes. Turn oven down to 300°. Slice the rectangles diagonally into 1/2-inch-thick slices. Place slices with cut-side down on ungreased baking sheets. Bake slices in 300° oven for another 5 to 10 minutes to make biscotti crisp.

Fran's Black Forrest Low-fat Brownie Swirl Cheesecake

Go ahead, have another slice.

Ingredients:
1 box (19 or 20 oz.) brownie mix recipe (replace eggs with Egg Beaters)
3 (8 oz.) containers low-fat or non-fat cream cheese at room temperature
1 cup sugar
1 teaspoon vanilla
1 (20 oz.) can light cherry pie filling

Preheat oven to 350°. Grease bottom of 9-inch springform pan. Prepare brownie mix as directed on box, replacing eggs with Egg Beaters. With an electric mixer, beat cream cheese, sugar, and vanilla until smooth. Pour cream cheese mixture into prepared springform pan. Drizzle brownie batter into cream cheese mixture and swirl gently with a spatula. Bake at 350° for 45 minutes until slightly firm. Edges should be slightly brown and cracks will form on top of cake. Cool on a rack to room temperature. Serve cheesecake topped with cherries.

Jennifer's Jack-O'-Lantern Parfait

Quick and easy—a real treat!

Ingredients:
1 1/2 cups skim milk
1 package (3.4 oz.) sugar-free instant butterscotch pudding mix
1 (15 oz.) can pumpkin
1 teaspoon pumpkin pie spice
1 (8 oz.) container fat-free whipped topping

Mix first four ingredients. Fold in whipped topping. Layer parfait into stemmed serving glasses, alternating layers with additional whipped topping. Refrigerate. Garnish with shaved dark chocolate.

Berry Tartlet
Berry, berry good

Ingredients:
1 cup hot water
1/2 cup canola oil
1 cup all-purpose flour
4 eggs, at room temperature
Pint of berries or berry mixture, in season or thawed
Confectioners' sugar for dusting, optional

Line nine cups of a large muffin tin with a piece of parchment paper in each cup. Place first two ingredients in thin saucepan. Bring to a rapid boil over medium-high heat. Reduce to low heat; add flour to liquid. Stir briskly until batter gathers into a ball. Remove from heat; allow to fully cool. Add eggs to mixture one at a time, beating until smooth. Spread batter into bottom and sides of each individual tin. Bake at 450° for 10 minutes. (Dough will puff while baking, but dip should remain.) Reduce to 400° for 20 to 25 minutes. Cool and fill with fresh berry mix. Dust with sugar.

Choffee
A tasty treat for chocoholics and coffee lovers alike

Ingredients:
1 single-serving package hot cocoa mix
6–8 oz. freshly brewed coffee

Empty hot cocoa mix into mug. Stir in hot coffee and enjoy.

Author's Before and After Photos

These photos represent my weight-loss journey based off the success principles in this book, and I hope they will help motivate you to achieve your weight-loss goals. If I can do it, so can you!

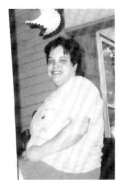

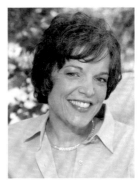

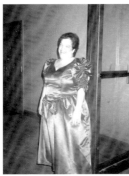

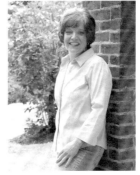

Courtesy Heidi Herholz, Evolutions Photography

Bibliography

1. As quoted in *The Edge* by Howard E. Ferguson. Revised edition 1990.

2. Foryet, J. P., G. K. Goodrick, and A. M. Gotto. 1981. "Limitations of behavioral treatment of obesity: Review and analysis." *Journal of Behavioral Medicine* 4: 159–173.

3. Fuhrman, Joel. 1995. *Fasting and Eating for Health* 8: 188.

Notes